DETAILS MYTHS AND FACTS ON HIV/AIDS

Updated causes, symptoms, side effects and therapy of hiv/aids.

By

Dr DOUGLAS JASON

DETAILS MYTHS AND FACTS ON HIV/AIDS

DETAILS MYTHS AND FACTS ON HIV/AIDS

Copyright © (DR DOUGLAS JASON) 2022. All rights reserved

Before this document is duplicated or reproduced in any manner, the publisher's consent must be gained.

Therefore, the contents within can neither be stored electronically, transferred, nor kept in a database. Neither in part nor in full can the document be copied, scanned, faxed, or retained without approval from the publisher or creator.

DETAILS MYTHS AND FACTS ON HIV/AIDS

DETAILS MYTHS AND FACTS ON HIV/AIDS

TABLE OF CONTENT

ABOUT THE AUTHOR

INTRODUCTION

DETAILS MYTHS AND FACTS ON HIV/AIDS

TABLE OF CONTENT

DETAILS MYTHS AND FACTS ON HIV/AIDS

Updated causes, symptoms, side effects and therapy of hiv/aids.

INTRODUCTION

CHAPTER 1
DEFINITION OF HIV AND AIDS.

CHAPTER 2.
THE CAUSES OF HIV AND AIDS.

CHAPTER 3
SYMPTOMS OF HIV AND AIDS.

CHAPTER 4

DETAILS MYTHS AND FACTS ON HIV/AIDS

Types of HIV Infections.

CHAPTER 5.
OPPORTUNISTIC INFECTIONS THAT SIGNATURE STAGE 3 HIV.

CHAPTER 6
discussed HIV-related health issues.

CHAPTER 7
Types of cancer connected to HIV.

CHAPTER 8
HOW TO AVOID HIV COMPLICATIONS.

CHAPTER 9
HOW TO DIAGNOSE HIV.

CHAPTER 10
HIV TREATMENT.

DETAILS MYTHS AND FACTS ON HIV/AIDS

CHAPTER 11
ANTIRETROVIRAL SIDE EFFECTS AND PREVENTIVE MECHANISMS

CONCLUSION

ABOUT THE AUTHOR

Dr. Douglas Jason is a certified dietician who has a strong passion for wellness and a big eagerness to help people all over the world. He uses healthy food, herbs, spices, and other useful tools to help mankind realize its overall goal of optimum health.

DETAILS MYTHS AND FACTS ON HIV/AIDS

DETAILS MYTHS AND FACTS ON HIV/AIDS

INTRODUCTION

The immune system is a target of HIV, which also modifies it, raising the risk and severity of other infections and disorders. Without treatment, the infection may develop to stage 3, sometimes known as HIV or AIDS.

Medical progress means that patients with HIV who have access to great healthcare and receive the right treatment are much less likely to progress to stage 3 of HIV or AIDS.

DETAILS MYTHS AND FACTS ON HIV/AIDS

The World Health Organization (WHO) and various other medical organizations have shown that many HIV-positive patients can control their illness and lead long, healthy lives.

The lifespan of an HIV-positive individual is now comparable to that of an HIV-negative person. This only holds, though, provided the patient consistently follows the doctor's instructions when undergoing

DETAILS MYTHS AND FACTS ON HIV/AIDS

antiretroviral therapy, a cocktail of medications.

Around 73% of adults and 54% of children with HIV received lifetime antiretroviral therapy as of 2020.

In this book, the causes, symptoms, and therapies of HIV and AIDS are discussed.

DETAILS MYTHS AND FACTS ON HIV/AIDS

CHAPTER 1

DEFINITION OF HIV AND AIDS.

Human immunodeficiency virus, or HIV, targets immune cells known as CD4 cells. These are different varieties of T cells, which are white blood cells that go throughout the body and look for infections, flaws, and abnormalities in other cells.

DETAILS MYTHS AND FACTS ON HIV/AIDS

HIV strives out and raids CD4 cells, using them to multiply the virus. As a a consequence, the cells are demolished, and the body's capacity to fight off additional infections and diseases is diminished.
Opportunistic infections and some cancers are more likely to occur as an outcome, as are their effects.

It is vital to keep in mind that some people with HIV might go for extended periods without showing any symptoms.

DETAILS MYTHS AND FACTS ON HIV/AIDS

Even though HIV is a lifelong affliction, various methods and treatments can stop the virus from spreading and the disease from worsening.

Describe AIDS.
Acquired immunodeficiency syndrome is referred to as AIDS. HIV has proceeded to this stage.

DETAILS MYTHS AND FACTS ON HIV/AIDS

A CD4 count of fewer than 200 cells per cubic millimeter is what medical professionals use to diagnose AIDS. A person may also be diagnosed with AIDS if they exhibit typical opportunistic ailments, related cancers, or both.

Without therapy, an HIV patient's immune system rapidly deteriorates, most likely resulting in stage 3 HIV. However, improvements in antiretroviral medications have reduced the frequency of this development.

DETAILS MYTHS AND FACTS ON HIV/AIDS

To be exact, there were 15,815 HIV-related deaths in the United States in 2019 and around 1.2 million people with HIV. Any reason could have caused these fatalities.

DETAILS MYTHS AND FACTS ON HIV/AIDS

CHAPTER 2.

THE CAUSES OF HIV AND AIDS.

HIV can circulate when bodily fluids containing the virus come into touch with a bodily barrier that is porous or when there are little tears in moist tissues in places like the genitals.

Specifically, HIV can disperse through of

DETAILS MYTHS AND FACTS ON HIV/AIDS

blood\ssemen
Premenstrual fluid
bodily fluids
urinary fluids
mother's milk
Because the virus cannot spread through saliva, for example, a person cannot get HIV through an open-mouthed kiss.

Anal or vaginal sex is one of the main methods of HIV transmission in the United States. When persons don't wear barrier protection, such

DETAILS MYTHS AND FACTS ON HIV/AIDS

as a condom, during sexual contact or don't take pre-exposure prophylaxis (PrEP), a medication designed to lower their risk of contracting HIV, it can lead to HIV transmission.

Another major factor in HIV transmission in the US is sharing injecting equipment.

HIV transmission to infants occurs less frequently during pregnancy,

DETAILS MYTHS AND FACTS ON HIV/AIDS

delivery, breastfeeding, and chest feeding.

Although the danger is very minimal when blood donations go through efficient screening, there is a chance of transmission through blood transfusions as well.

Untransmittable = undetectable
Only liquids with a specific level of HIV can transfer the virus. HIV cannot spread from one person to another if the person has

DETAILS MYTHS AND FACTS ON HIV/AIDS

undetectable levels of the virus. Even though there is essentially no danger of transmission during sex, it is unknown whether there is a risk reduction while sharing injection medication equipment.

Additionally, the danger of transmission is much diminished—though still present—during pregnancy and childbirth.

The idea that HIV is not transmittable at undetectable levels

DETAILS MYTHS AND FACTS ON HIV/AIDS

is sometimes expressed as a shorthand: U=U.

When the level of the virus in the body is so low that a blood test cannot detect it, doctors consider HIV to be undetectable.

A person must consistently obtain successful treatment and strictly adhere to the suggested treatment plan to reach undetectable levels. Typically, daily drug administration is required.

DETAILS MYTHS AND FACTS ON HIV/AIDS

HIV can still be present in undetectable quantities, and ongoing blood testing is essential to preserving this status.

development into AIDS
The likelihood that HIV will develop into AIDS varies greatly from person to person and depends on a variety of factors, including:

DETAILS MYTHS AND FACTS ON HIV/AIDS

age and a person's body's capacity to fight HIV
access to high-quality medical treatment
additional infections are present
a person's genetic susceptibility to particular HIV strains, some of which are drug-resistant

DETAILS MYTHS AND FACTS ON HIV/AIDS

CHAPTER 3

SYMPTOMS OF HIV AND AIDS.

The more severe symptoms of HIV are typically caused by secondary illnesses with bacteria, viruses, fungi, or parasites.

Early HIV symptoms
After getting the infection, some HIV-positive individuals go months or even years without showing any

DETAILS MYTHS AND FACTS ON HIV/AIDS

symptoms. In part as a result of this, 13% of Americans who have HIV are unaware that they do.

There is still a substantial risk of transmission even though a person with no symptoms may be less likely to seek medical attention. To ensure that everyone is informed of their HIV status, specialists advise routine testing.

While this is going on, almost two-thirds of HIV patients experience flu-

DETAILS MYTHS AND FACTS ON HIV/AIDS

like symptoms 2-4 weeks after getting the virus. Acute retroviral syndrome is a term used to describe these symptoms as a whole.

HIV can present with early signs like:

a fever chills, especially at night, sweating, enlarged glands, or swollen lymph nodes
a widespread rash, weakness, and pain, especially joint pain
body pains and a sore throat

DETAILS MYTHS AND FACTS ON HIV/AIDS

These signs and symptoms are the outcomes of the immune system battling the illness. Anyone who exhibits several of these signs and may have acquired HIV during the last two to six weeks ought to get tested.

Some HIV symptoms are gender-specific. Learn more about the symptoms that affect men and women.
in

DETAILS MYTHS AND FACTS ON HIV/AIDS

DETAILS MYTHS AND FACTS ON HIV/AIDS

CHAPTER 4

Types of HIV Infections.

1. **HIV symptomatic**
Many patients may not experience any HIV symptoms for years after the acute retroviral syndrome symptoms subside.

The virus develops and harms the immune system and organs even though individuals feel fine and seem to be in good health. This gradual process can last for ten

DETAILS MYTHS AND FACTS ON HIV/AIDS

years or longer if the patient does not take medication that stops the virus from replicating. However, other people might advance more quickly.

Antiretroviral medication can halt this process and completely eradicate the infection.

.

Secondly, advanced HIV infection If an individual with HIV does not receive appropriate treatment, the virus erodes the body's defenses

DETAILS MYTHS AND FACTS ON HIV/AIDS

against infection, leaving it vulnerable to life-threatening diseases.

A clinician can identify stage 3 HIV when CD4 cells are substantially reduced and there are less than 200 cells per cubic millimeter.

A clinician can recognize stage 3 HIV by looking for certain opportunistic illnesses caused by bacteria, viruses, fungi, or mycobacteria.

DETAILS MYTHS AND FACTS ON HIV/AIDS

However, a person with AIDS can control, prevent, and treat significant consequences by taking additional drugs in addition to HIV treatment.

A person with HIV may never reach stage 3 of the infection if they receive adequate therapy. A person can regain some of their immune function with treatment, which will aid in preventing dangerous infections.

Cancer and opportunistic infections

DETAILS MYTHS AND FACTS ON HIV/AIDS

HIV stage 3 impairs the body's capacity to fight off a variety of infections, their related consequences, and many cancers.

Many infections can be controlled with the current treatments. If an HIV-positive individual does not receive treatment, latent infections that previously caused little to no health issues could become dangerous. Opportunistic diseases are what doctors refer to as.

DETAILS MYTHS AND FACTS ON HIV/AIDS

CHAPTER 5.

OPPORTUNISTIC INFECTIONS THAT SIGNATURE STAGE 3 HIV.

The following opportunistic conditions can alert a physician that a patient has stage 3 HIV:

1. Candidiasis is a fungal illness that generally affects the skin and nails, but in AIDS patients, it frequently causes major issues with

DETAILS MYTHS AND FACTS ON HIV/AIDS

the esophagus and lower respiratory system.

2.) Coccidioidomycosis: This condition is brought on by inhaling the fungus Coccidioides limits. In healthy individuals, a doctor would call this infection valley fever.

3.) Cryptococcosis: This condition is caused by the fungus Cryptococcus neoformans. Although it can affect any region of the body, pneumonia is typically brought on by fungus entering the lungs. Additionally, the brain may swell as a result.

DETAILS MYTHS AND FACTS ON HIV/AIDS

(4.) Cryptosporidiosis: This protozoan parasite infection can cause extreme stomach pains and persistent, watery diarrhea. Cytomegalovirus disease (CMV): CMV is a virus that can cause several illnesses, such as encephalitis, pneumonia, and gastroenteritis. People with AIDS should be especially concerned about CMV retinitis. This is an infection of the retina at the back of the eye, which results in vision loss that cannot be reversed. A medical emergency has arisen.

DETAILS MYTHS AND FACTS ON HIV/AIDS

(5.) Herpes: Herpes simplex virus infection causes this condition (HSV). When persons engage in anal or vaginal sex without utilizing barrier contraception, such as a condom, this virus typically spreads. Additionally, it might spread during vaginal delivery. A doctor might advise a cesarean delivery for a woman who has genital herpes and is about to give birth. As a result, there is a considerably lesser chance that the newborn may contract HSV.

6. Histoplasmosis: In persons with advanced HIV, this fungal infection

DETAILS MYTHS AND FACTS ON HIV/AIDS

causes severe, pneumonia-like symptoms. Additionally, histoplasmosis has the potential to spread and progress, impacting organs beyond the respiratory system.

7.) Tuberculosis (TB) is brought on by the bacterium Mycobacterium. When an infected individual sneeze, coughs or speaks, the germs can spread through the air. A serious lung infection, weight loss, a fever, and exhaustion are a few of the warning signs and symptoms. It can circulate to other organs, including the brain.

DETAILS MYTHS AND FACTS ON HIV/AIDS

Mycobacterium avium and Mycobacterium kansasii are two types of mycobacteria that are normally present and typically do not create many issues. However, these infections can spread throughout the body and result in life-threatening health problems in people who have HIV, particularly in the latter stages of the disease.

9.) Recurrent pneumonia: Although a variety of microorganisms can cause pneumonia, Streptococcus pneumonia bacteria may be among the most harmful for those who have

DETAILS MYTHS AND FACTS ON HIV/AIDS

HIV. Every person with HIV should obtain the available vaccine against this bacteria.

(10.) Pneumocystis jirovecii pneumonia: In persons with weakened immune systems, such as some HIV-positive individuals, an infection with this fungus can result in dyspnea, a dry cough, and a high temperature.

(11) Chronic intestinal isosporiasis: This condition develops when the parasite Isospora belli enters the body through tainted food or water and causes vomiting, diarrhea, weight

DETAILS MYTHS AND FACTS ON HIV/AIDS

loss, headaches, and abdominal pain.

(12.) Salmonella septicemia that recurs: Salmonella bacteria can circulate and overwhelm the immune system when they enter the body, typically through contaminated food or water, resulting in nausea, diarrhea, and vomiting. A physician might make the diagnosis of Salmonella septicemia in this situation.

(13.)Toxoplasmosis is caused by the parasite Toxoplasma gondii, which lives inside warm-blooded animals like cats and rats and is

DETAILS MYTHS AND FACTS ON HIV/AIDS

found in their feces. Humans who consume contaminated food or breathe in contaminated dust become infected with toxoplasmosis. It may result in severe symptoms that affect the testes, colon, liver, pancreas, liver, lungs, retina, heart, and liver. Wear gloves and thoroughly wash your hands after changing the cat's litter to lower your risk of getting toxoplasmosis.

DETAILS MYTHS AND FACTS ON HIV/AIDS

CHAPTER 6

discussed HIV-related health issues.

Complications that an individual with advanced HIV or an opportunistic infection may encounter include:

(1) HIV-related encephalopathy: HIV can cause encephalopathy or brain inflammation. The underlying mechanisms are not fully understood by physicians.

DETAILS MYTHS AND FACTS ON HIV/AIDS

PML, or progressive multifocal leukoencephalopathy, is caused by the John Cunningham virus infection. This virus is widespread and typically rests latent in the kidneys. The John Cunningham virus affects the brain and causes PML in people with compromised immune systems, which may be brought on by HIV or drugs used to treat multiple sclerosis. It may be fatal, resulting in paralysis, and impairing cognitive function.

3. Wasting syndrome: Wasting syndrome is a condition in which an individual unintentionally loses 10%

DETAILS MYTHS AND FACTS ON HIV/AIDS

of their muscle mass due to weakness, diarrhea, or a fever. Fat loss could contribute to some of the weight loss.

DETAILS MYTHS AND FACTS ON HIV/AIDS

CHAPTER 7

Types of cancer connected to HIV.

A person with HIV may be more susceptible to some cancers, including lymphoma.

A kind of cancer that includes the development of aberrant blood vessels is brought on by the Kaposi sarcoma herpesvirus (KSHV), also known as human herpesvirus 8.

DETAILS MYTHS AND FACTS ON HIV/AIDS

Anywhere throughout the body, they can develop.

If cancer spreads to vital organs like the intestines or lymph nodes, it may be exceedingly hazardous. Characteristic flat or raised solid, purplish, pink, brown, or black patches can be identified by a doctor.

In addition, HIV is strongly associated with both Hodgkin's and non-Hodgkin's lymphoma. The lymph nodes and lymphoid tissues are affected by these malignancies.

DETAILS MYTHS AND FACTS ON HIV/AIDS

VIRGINIA CANCER

A female with HIV should also get routine screenings for cervical cancer. According to a new study, women who are HIV-positive are more likely to get cervical cancer than women who are HIV-negative. Early diagnosis helps prevent the progression of the disease.

DETAILS MYTHS AND FACTS ON HIV/AIDS

CHAPTER 8

HOW TO AVOID HIV COMPLICATIONS.

Eliminating problems
The key to extending the life of someone with late-stage HIV is prevention.

With HIV drugs, it's critical to control viral load while also taking extra safety measures, such as:

DETAILS MYTHS AND FACTS ON HIV/AIDS

using condoms to avoid more sexually transmitted diseases (STIs)

getting immunized against probable opportunistic diseases

recognizing and reducing exposure to any environmental factors that could cause infection, such as using gloves when changing cat litter, avoiding foods with a high risk of contamination, such as raw seed sprouts, unpasteurized dairy products, and unfiltered tap water in some countries, and consulting a doctor about any necessary vaccinations and ways to reduce exposure to pathogens at work.

DETAILS MYTHS AND FACTS ON HIV/AIDS

Opportunistic infections can be treated with antibiotics, antifungals, and anti-parasitic medications.

There are a lot of HIV-related myths out there. These are damaging and derogatory.

The following actions or conduct won't result in virus transmission:

extending a hand
kissing, sneezing, embracing, and touching unbroken skin
Using a bathroom with an HIV-positive person

DETAILS MYTHS AND FACTS ON HIV/AIDS

exchange of towels
Sharing utensils, performing mouth-to-mouth resuscitation, or handling an HIV-positive person's saliva, tears, excrement, or urine

CHAPTER 9

HOW TO DIAGNOSE HIV.

According to data, 13% of HIV-positive individuals in the United

DETAILS MYTHS AND FACTS ON HIV/AIDS

States alone are not aware of their condition.

For a person's health and well-being, knowing their HIV status is essential since it can help them get the necessary treatment early and avoid consequences.

A person's blood can be tested by medical professionals for HIV antibodies. Before declaring the blood to be positive, they will retest it.

DETAILS MYTHS AND FACTS ON HIV/AIDS

There are additional kits for use at home.

Using the most recent HIV testing technologies, HIV can be found in less than two weeks.

People who have recognized risk factors ought to get tested more frequently.

A fast test is available to anyone who suspects they may be at risk of catching HIV. The test provider typically advises getting another test

DETAILS MYTHS AND FACTS ON HIV/AIDS

within a few weeks if this results in a negative result.

The following are the several HIV test types:

As early as 10 days after exposure, nucleic acid amplification tests, often known as NATs, are capable of detecting HIV.
As early as 18 days after exposure, an antigen/antibody blood test can identify HIV in a blood sample.
Antibody tests, which are the most common quick testing and self-tests,

DETAILS MYTHS AND FACTS ON HIV/AIDS

can find HIV antibodies as early as 21 days after exposure.

A person should discuss post-exposure prophylaxis (PEP), a preventive therapy, with a healthcare provider if they believe they may have been exposed to HIV during the last 72 hours.

A length of time known as the wind period exists between HIV exposure and the point at which a test can identify it. The window period, however, may differ depending on the individual and the HIV detection test used.

DETAILS MYTHS AND FACTS ON HIV/AIDS

CHAPTER 10

HIV TREATMENT.

HIV cannot be cured, although certain medications can halt its spread.

Antiretroviral medications can lessen the likelihood of transmission. They can also increase a person's quality of life and lengthen their lifespan.

DETAILS MYTHS AND FACTS ON HIV/AIDS

Many HIV-positive patients lead long, healthy lives. The majority of patients tolerate these drugs well, and they are getting more and more effective. One pill a day may be all that is required.

HIV drugs and treatment options.

Emergency HIV medications: PEP Anyone who thinks they may have been exposed to the virus within the previous 72 hours ought to talk to a doctor about post-exposure prophylaxis (PEP).

DETAILS MYTHS AND FACTS ON HIV/AIDS

If PEP is taken as soon as possible after the probable exposure, it may be able to stop the infection.

After taking PEP for 28 days, a patient has their HIV status checked by a doctor.

Although PEP is often effective, it is still vital to follow safe injection procedures and barrier protection when taking PEP.

Antiretroviral medications

DETAILS MYTHS AND FACTS ON HIV/AIDS

Antiretroviral drugs are used to treat HIV because they fight the infection and stop the virus's spread.

Highly active antiretroviral therapy, often known as combination antiretroviral therapy, is typically administered to patients. The method may be referred to as HAART or cART, respectively.

several kinds of antiretrovirals, such as:

Protease blockers

DETAILS MYTHS AND FACTS ON HIV/AIDS

HIV requires the enzyme protease to reproduce. HIV cannot replicate because protease inhibitors bind to the enzyme and stop it from working.

Types consist of:

cobicistat with atazanavir (Evotaz)
ritonavir with lopinavir (Kaletra)
Integrase inhibitors darunavir and cobicistat (Prezcobix)
Integrase inhibitors prevent HIV from infecting T cells by inhibiting the integrase enzyme. Doctors frequently recommend them as the

DETAILS MYTHS AND FACTS ON HIV/AIDS

first line of treatment due to their efficacy and few adverse effects.

Among the integrase inhibitors are:

Raltegravir and dolutegravir (Tivicay) (Isentress)
Reverse transcriptase inhibitors for nucleosides and nucleotides
These medications, often known as NRTIs or "nukes," prevent HIV from replicating.

Types consist of:

DETAILS MYTHS AND FACTS ON HIV/AIDS

Emtricitabine (Emtriva), abacavir (Ziagen), lamivudine and zidovudine (Combivir), and tenofovir disoproxil (Viread)
inhibitors of non-nucleoside reverse transcriptase
Additionally, the NNRTIs increase the difficulty of HIV replication.

Types consist of:

efavirenz (Sustiva), doravirine (Pifeltro), and etravirine (Intelence) Agonists of the chemokine coreceptor nevirapine (Viramune)

DETAILS MYTHS AND FACTS ON HIV/AIDS

These medicines stop HIV from infecting cells. However, because they are not as effective as certain other medications, American doctors rarely prescribe them.
Entrance blockers
HIV cannot enter T cells due to entry inhibitors. If HIV cannot penetrate these cells, it cannot replicate. In the US, entry inhibitors are likewise not frequent.

Antiretroviral medication combinations are frequently beneficial for patients, and the ideal

DETAILS MYTHS AND FACTS ON HIV/AIDS

combination depends on aspects that are unique to each patient.

HIV therapy entails taking medications regularly for the rest of one's life.

DETAILS MYTHS AND FACTS ON HIV/AIDS

CHAPTER 11

ANTIRETROVIRAL SIDE EFFECTS AND PREVENTIVE MECHANISMS

Although the adverse effects of each class of antiretrovirals vary, a few typical ones are as follows:

nausea\sfatigue
diarrhea\sheadaches\srashes

DETAILS MYTHS AND FACTS ON HIV/AIDS

Alternative or complementary medicine

Many HIV patients experiment with supplementary, alternative, or herbal treatments. There is no proof that these are efficient, though.

Before taking any mineral or vitamin supplements, it is vital to discuss them with a healthcare provider because some natural items may interfere with HIV medications.

PREVENTIONS

DETAILS MYTHS AND FACTS ON HIV/AIDS

The following methods can be used to avoid HIV contact.

Using PrEP and barrier protection When having anal, vaginal, or oral intercourse, using condoms or other barrier protection, such as dental dams, can significantly lower a person's risk of getting HIV and other STIs.

When having insertive vaginal sex with a partner who has a penis, transgender women and non-binary people who were born male and

DETAILS MYTHS AND FACTS ON HIV/AIDS

have undergone vaginoplasty are at risk of contracting HIV.

The Preventive Services Task Force encourages clinicians to only authorize PrEP for those with recent negative HIV tests in their 2019 guidelines.

They also approve a PrEP formulation that combines emtricitabine and tenofovir disoproxil fumarate. They encourage PrEP users to take it once daily.

DETAILS MYTHS AND FACTS ON HIV/AIDS

Tenofovir alafenamide and emtricitabine, a second medication combination, have also received FDA approval for use as PrEP.

employing safe injection techniques One important way that HIV is spread is through intravenous drug usage. HIV and other infections, such as hepatitis C, can be spread via sharing needles and other drug-related supplies.

Any drug user who injects himself should use a clean, unused needle.

DETAILS MYTHS AND FACTS ON HIV/AIDS

Programs for addiction rehabilitation and needle exchange can help lower the prevalence of HIV.

avoiding contact with pertinent bodily fluids
Reduce contact with blood, semen, vaginal secretions, and other bodily fluids that the virus can be present in to lessen the chance of HIV exposure.

The risk of infection can also be decreased by often and thoroughly

DETAILS MYTHS AND FACTS ON HIV/AIDS

cleaning the skin after it has come into touch with bodily fluids.

When exposure to these fluids is likely, healthcare personnel use gloves, masks, protective eyewear, face shields, and gowns to avoid transmission and adhere to established protocols.

Pregnancy
While some antiretrovirals can be harmful to the fetus while a woman is pregnant, transmission can be

DETAILS MYTHS AND FACTS ON HIV/AIDS

stopped with an efficient, well-managed treatment strategy.

If the person with HIV maintains the illness adequately, vaginal births are feasible.

The virus might also be able to spread through breast milk. Regardless of viral load or use of antiretrovirals, the Centers for Disease Control and Prevention (CDC) do not advise breastfeeding or chestfeeding.

DETAILS MYTHS AND FACTS ON HIV/AIDS

It's crucial to completely go over all the possibilities with a healthcare practitioner.

Education
To prevent HIV exposure, it is essential to understand the risk factors.

Having HIV/AIDS
Many HIV-positive persons have full, active lives. However, it is crucial to use the following tactics because of the possibility of immune system harm.

DETAILS MYTHS AND FACTS ON HIV/AIDS

maintaining a drug schedule
It is crucial to take HIV medication as directed; skipping even a few doses could make the treatment less effective.

A person should create a daily medication schedule that works with their schedule and treatment plan.

Sometimes side effects make it difficult for patients to follow their treatment regimens. Contact a healthcare provider if any adverse effect is challenging to manage.

DETAILS MYTHS AND FACTS ON HIV/AIDS

They may propose switching to a medication that is better tolerated as well as other treatment-related modifications.

enhancing general health
The idea is to take precautions to be healthy and prevent infections. People with HIV should engage in regular exercise, consume a balanced diet, and abstain from harmful behaviors like smoking.

Preventing exposure to germs that cause infection is extremely crucial.

DETAILS MYTHS AND FACTS ON HIV/AIDS

This can entail refraining from consuming unpasteurized meals and undercooked meats as well as avoiding contact with cat litter and animal excrement.

It's also important to wash your hands thoroughly and frequently.

Antiretrovirals lessen the necessity for the aforementioned precautions overall.

communicating with doctors
Since HIV is a lifetime condition, it is significant to routinely consult with a

DETAILS MYTHS AND FACTS ON HIV/AIDS

medical team to make sure that the patient's regimen is appropriate for their age and any coexisting conditions. The treatment plan will be reviewed by the team and modified as necessary.

promotion of mental health
There is a great deal of stigma surrounding HIV and AIDS, as well as many myths. As a result, a person might experience persecution, loneliness, or exclusion.

DETAILS MYTHS AND FACTS ON HIV/AIDS

An HIV diagnosis can be extremely upsetting, and anxiety or sadness are frequent feelings. A trusted medical or mental health expert might be consulted for assistance.

The CDC offers a list of programs that might assist people in coping with prejudice and stigma and in obtaining extra support.

CONCLUSION

DETAILS MYTHS AND FACTS ON HIV/AIDS

HIV is a viral illness that weakens the immune system's capacity. A person with HIV can live a long, normal life if they have access to quality healthcare and take antiretroviral drugs, thanks to advancements in therapy.

Some physiological fluids, including blood, vaginal secretions, and semen, can spread HIV. Sharing needles and engaging in sexual activity without utilizing barrier protection or taking PrEP are the most prevalent methods of transmission in the United States.

DETAILS MYTHS AND FACTS ON HIV/AIDS

A person has an undetectable viral load if the levels of HIV in their body are so low that a test cannot detect them. The virus cannot infect someone else in this situation. An individual can accomplish this by using antiretrovirals.

HIV can advance to stage 3 HIV, or AIDS, if a person with the condition is not treated, potentially because they are unaware that they have the virus.

DETAILS MYTHS AND FACTS ON HIV/AIDS

A person with AIDS is more vulnerable to several infections and other potentially serious health problems.

HIV can occasionally go years without causing any symptoms or only create mild symptoms that are simple to confuse with the flu. Anyone in the U.S. who thinks they may have recently been exposed to HIV can find the closest testing center here.

DETAILS MYTHS AND FACTS ON HIV/AIDS

www.ingramcontent.com/pod-product-compliance
Lightning Source LLC
Chambersburg PA
CBHW070302220526
45465CB00004B/1712